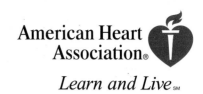

American Heart
Association®

Learn and Live SM

HEARTSAVER® AED

STUDENT WORKBOOK

ISBN 0-87493-467-2

Workbook Contents

Student CD Contents

CONTENTS

Considerations for International Readers

The following table is intended for international participants of this course. It is meant to help explain materials in this course that may be relevant only to those in the United States. For more specific information about your local practices and organizations, please contact your instructor.

Page 5	In the section **Actions for Compressions**, please note the following metric conversion: 1½ to 2 inches = 4 to 5 cm
Page 17	In the section **Using a Mask**, the Occupational Safety and Health Administration (OSHA) is referenced. OSHA is a US agency. Please contact your local authority about the safety and health standards for your workplace.
Page 27	In the section **Steps for Using an AED**, AED training information specific to the United States is given. Please consult your instructor for more information about AED training in your area.
Page 45	In the section **Access to Emergency Medical Service**, a telephone number is given for Poison Control in the United States. Please consult your instructor about the important emergency response numbers in your area.
Page 47	In the **Conclusion**, there are references to the American Heart Association's courses and contact information. For information most relevant to your area, please consult your instructor.
Page 48	In the **Compression depth** row of the table referring to Adult CPR, please note the following metric conversion: 1½ to 2 inches = 4 to 5 cm

Introduction

Course Goal

The American Heart Association designed the Heartsaver AED Course to prepare a wide variety of people who, as first responders,

- May need to perform cardiopulmonary resuscitation (CPR) in the workplace or similar settings
- May need to use an automated external defibrillator (AED)
- May need to help someone who is choking
- Want or need a course completion card

This student workbook includes information you need to give CPR in a safe, timely, and effective manner to an adult, child, or infant. It also provides information on using an AED for adults and children over 1 year of age.

The Importance of CPR

Heart attack, drowning, electric shock, and other problems may cause a victim's heart to stop pumping blood. This is called cardiac arrest.

Studies show that effective CPR right away improves survival from cardiac arrest. Most cardiac arrests happen outside the hospital, where bystander CPR is really important.

You can make a difference, and the first step is learning CPR. You never know when you might need to use the CPR skills you learn for someone you know or even one of your loved ones.

Who Should Take This Course

We created this course for anyone who needs to learn CPR, including corporate and retail employees, security, law enforcement, health and fitness staff, and anyone who needs a course completion card in CPR and AED.

How This Course Is Organized

You will learn CPR basics through this student workbook and the video for the course. You will have a chance to practice many times while the video guides you. When you are not practicing with the video, you may watch the video, watch the other students practice, or follow along in your student workbook.

During the course you will practice some skills. After you correctly demonstrate the skills taught in the course, you will receive a Heartsaver AED course completion card.

Using This Student Workbook

This student workbook is a classroom textbook. You should use this workbook in the following ways:

When	Then you should
Before the course	• Read this student workbook and look at the pictures on each page. • Answer the review questions at the end of each section.
During the course	• Use this workbook to help you understand the important information and skills taught in the course.
After the course	• Review the skills frequently. Look at the practice sheets in the workbook. This will help you remember the steps of CPR and AED use, and you'll be ready if there is an emergency.

Student Workbook Organization

This student workbook contains the following sections:

- Adult CPR
- Child CPR
- Use of a Mask—Adult/Child
- Adult/Child Choking
- Using AEDs
- Infant CPR
- Use of a Mask—Infant
- Infant Choking
- Phoning for Help

Review Questions

Many of the sections in this workbook include review questions for you to answer. Try to answer the questions as you review the book before class. Your instructor will give you the answers during class.

Using the Student CD

More information is available on the CD (included with this workbook). Look in the Heartsaver AED section.

You should use the student CD in the following ways:

When	Then you should
Before the course	• Watch the video clips. This will help you learn the important points and prepare for practice during the course.
After the course	• View the video clips after class as a review. • Review the reference materials and other information on the CD.

See the list of CD contents following the table of contents in this student workbook.

CD Icon

The CD icon will help you as you use this student workbook.

Icon	Meaning
	Check the student CD for more information about this topic.

Reminders

Your student workbook includes CPR and AED reminders. Keep them handy to help you remember the steps of CPR and how to use an AED.

How Often Training Is Needed

Review your student workbook, student CD, and CPR and AED reminders often to keep your skills fresh. You need to retake this course every 2 years to get a new course completion card.

Adult CPR

What You Will Learn By the end of this section you should be able to give CPR to an adult.

Ages for Adult CPR Adult CPR is for victims 8 years of age and older.

Overview

If you know *when* to phone your emergency response number (or 911) and *how* to give compressions and breaths, your actions may save a life. In this course you will learn the basic steps of CPR first. Then you will put these steps together in order.

There are basic steps in giving CPR:

- Doing compressions
- Giving breaths that make the chest rise

Compressions

One of the most important parts of adult CPR is compressions. When you give compressions, you pump blood to the brain and heart. You will learn more about where compressions fit in the sequence of CPR later.

Actions for Compressions

Follow these steps to give compressions to adults:

Step	Action
1	Kneel at the victim's side.
2	Make sure the victim is lying on his back on a firm, flat surface. If the victim is lying facedown, carefully roll him onto his back.
3	Quickly move or remove clothes from the front of the chest that will get in the way of doing compressions and using an AED.
4	Put the heel of one hand on the center of the victim's chest between the nipples (Figure 1A). Put the heel of your other hand on top of the first hand (Figure 1B).
5	Push straight down on the chest 1½ to 2 inches with each compression. Push hard and fast.
6	Push at a rate of 100 compressions a minute.
7	After each compression, release pressure on the chest to let it come back to its normal position.

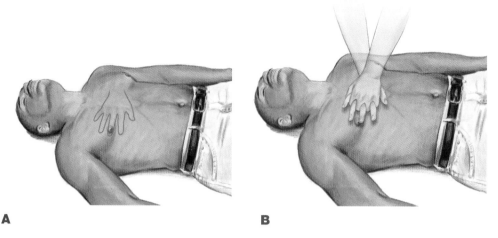

A   **B**

Figure 1. Chest compressions. **A,** Put the heel of one hand on the center of the chest between the nipples. **B,** Put the other hand on top of the first hand.

> ### *Important*
>
> These things are important to remember when doing CPR:
>
> - Push hard and push fast.
> - Push at a rate of 100 times a minute.
> - After each compression, release pressure on the chest to let it come back to its normal position.

Open the Airway

When giving CPR you must give the victim breaths that make the chest rise. Before giving breaths, you must open the airway with the head tilt–chin lift.

Performing the Head Tilt–Chin Lift

Follow these steps to perform a head tilt–chin lift:

Step	Action
1	Tilt the head by pushing back on the forehead.
2	Lift the chin by putting your fingers on the bony part of the chin. Do not press the soft tissues of the neck or under the chin (Figure 2).
3	Lift the chin to move the jaw forward.

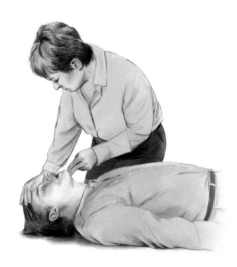

Figure 2. Open the airway with a head tilt–chin lift.

Giving Breaths

Your breaths give oxygen to someone who cannot breathe on his own.

Actions for Giving Breaths

Follow these steps to give breaths:

Step	Action
1	Hold the airway open with a head tilt–chin lift (Figure 2).
2	Pinch the nose closed.
3	Take a normal breath and cover the victim's mouth with your mouth, creating an airtight seal.
4	Give 2 breaths (blow for 1 second each). Watch for chest rise as you give each breath (Figure 3).

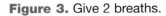

Figure 3. Give 2 breaths.

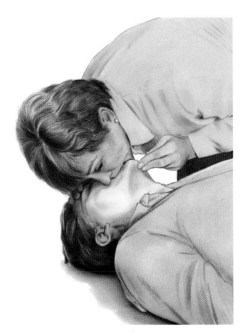

Compressions and Breaths	When you give CPR, you do sets of 30 compressions and 2 breaths. Try not to interrupt chest compressions for more than a few seconds. For example, don't take too long to give breaths or use the AED.

Putting It All Together	You have learned compressions and breaths for an adult. To put it all together in the right order, follow these steps.

Make Sure the Scene Is Safe	Before you give CPR, make sure the scene is safe for you and the victim (Figure 4). For example, make sure there is no traffic in the area that could injure you. You do not want to become a victim yourself.

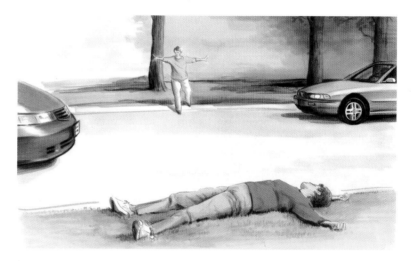

Figure 4. Make sure the scene is safe.

Check for Response	Check to see if the victim responds before giving CPR. Kneel at the victim's side. Tap the victim and shout, "Are you OK?" (Figure 5).

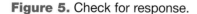

Figure 5. Check for response.

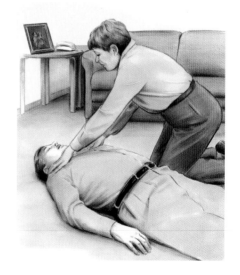

Get Help

If the victim does not respond, it is important to get help on the way as soon as possible. Follow these steps to call for help:

Step	Action
1	If the victim does not respond, yell for help. If someone comes, send that person to phone your emergency response number (or 911) and get the AED if available.
2	If no one comes, leave the victim to phone your emergency response number (or 911) and get the AED if available (Figure 6). Return to the victim and start the steps of CPR.

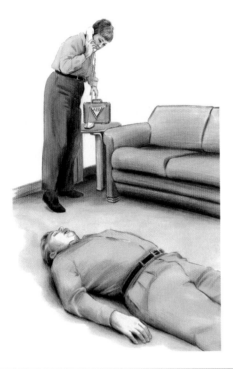

Figure 6. Phone your emergency response number (or 911) and get the AED if available.

Check Breathing

Once you have checked the victim for a response, you must check to see if the victim is breathing normally.

Step	Action
1	Open the victim's airway with a head tilt–chin lift.
2	Check to see if the victim is breathing normally (take at least 5 seconds but no more than 10 seconds) (Figure 7). • Put your ear next to the victim's mouth and nose. • **Look** to see if the chest rises. • **Listen** for breaths. • **Feel** for breaths on your cheek.

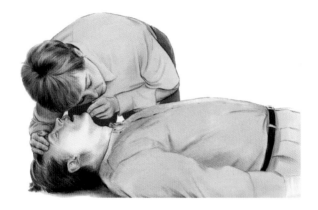

Figure 7. Look, listen, and feel for normal breathing.

Special Situations

Gasps Are Not Breaths

In the first few minutes after sudden cardiac arrest, a victim may only gasp.

Gasping is *not* breathing.

> **Important**
>
> If the victim gasps when you open the airway to check breathing, continue the steps of CPR. The victim is likely to need all the steps of CPR.

If the First Breath Does Not Go In

If you give a victim a breath and it does not go in, you will need to re-open the airway with a head tilt–chin lift before giving the second breath. After you give 2 breaths, you will give 30 compressions. You will repeat the sets of 30 compressions and 2 breaths until the AED arrives, the victim starts to move, or trained help takes over. Trained help could be someone whose job is taking care of people who are ill or injured such as an EMS responder, nurse, or doctor.

Side Position

If the victim is breathing normally but is not responding, roll the victim to his side and wait for trained help to take over (Figure 8). If the victim stops moving again, you will need to start the steps of CPR from the beginning.

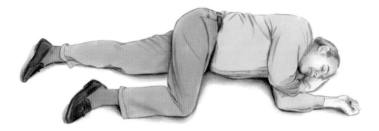

Figure 8. Side position.

Summary of Steps for Adult CPR

The following table summarizes the steps for adult CPR:

Step	Action
1	Make sure the scene is safe.
2	Make sure the victim is lying on his back on a firm, flat surface. If the victim is lying facedown, carefully roll him onto his back.
3	Kneel at the victim's side. Tap and shout to see if the victim responds.
4	If the victim does not respond, yell for help. • If someone comes, send that person to phone your emergency response number (or 911) and get the AED if available. • If no one comes, leave the victim to phone your emergency response number (or 911) and get the AED if available. After you answer all the dispatcher's questions, return to the victim and start the steps of CPR.
5	Open the airway with a head tilt–chin lift.
6	Check to see if the victim is breathing normally (take at least 5 seconds but no more than 10 seconds). • Put your ear next to the victim's mouth and nose. • **Look** to see if the chest rises. • **Listen** for breaths. • **Feel** for breaths on your cheek.
7	If there is no normal breathing, give 2 breaths (1 second each). Watch for chest rise as you give each breath.
8	Quickly move or remove clothes from the front of the chest that will get in the way of doing compressions and using an AED.
9	Give 30 compressions at a rate of 100 a minute and then give 2 breaths. After each compression, release pressure on the chest to let it come back to its normal position.
10	Keep giving sets of 30 compressions and 2 breaths until the AED arrives, the victim starts to move, or trained help takes over.

Review Questions

1. The correct rate for giving compressions is _____ compressions a minute.
2. For adult CPR you give sets of _____ compressions and _____ breaths.
3. When giving CPR how long should each breath take?
   a. 1 second
   b. 3 seconds
   c. 4 seconds

Child CPR

What You Will Learn   By the end of this section you should be able to give CPR to a child.

Ages for Child CPR   For purposes of this course, a child is 1 to 8 years of age.

Overview   Although some steps for giving CPR to an adult and child are similar, there are a few differences:

- When to phone your emergency response number (or 911)
- Amount of air for breaths
- Depth of compressions
- Number of hands for compressions

When to Phone Your Emergency Response Number (or 911)   If you are alone, do 5 sets of 30 compressions and 2 breaths *before* leaving the victim to phone your emergency response number (or 911). This is different from adult CPR, where you phone first.

Amount of Air for Breaths   Breaths are very important for children who do not respond. When giving breaths to children, be sure to open the airway and give breaths that make the chest rise, just as for adults. For small children you will not need to use the same amount of air for breaths as for larger children or adults. However, each breath should still make the chest rise.

Depth of Compressions

When you push on a child's chest, press straight down ⅓ to ½ the depth of the chest (Figure 9).

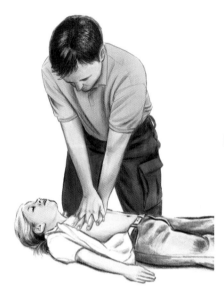

Figure 9. Two-handed chest compressions.

Number of Hands for Compressions

You may need to use only 1 hand for compressions for very small children (Figure 10). Whether you use 1 hand or 2 hands, it is important to be sure to push straight down ⅓ to ½ the depth of the chest.

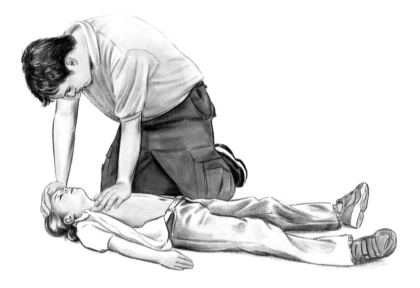

Figure 10. One-handed chest compressions.

Summary of Steps for Child CPR

The following table shows the steps for giving CPR to a child 1 to 8 years of age.

Step	Action
1	Make sure the scene is safe.
2	Make sure the victim is lying on her back on a firm, flat surface. If the victim is lying facedown, carefully roll her onto her back.
3	Kneel at the victim's side. Tap and shout to see if the victim responds.
4	If the victim does not respond, yell for help. • If someone comes, send that person to phone your emergency response number (or 911) and get the AED if available. • If no one comes, stay with the child and start the steps of CPR.
5	Open the airway with a head tilt–chin lift.
6	Check to see if the victim is breathing (take at least 5 seconds but no more than 10 seconds). • Put your ear next to the victim's mouth and nose. • **Look** to see if the chest rises. • **Listen** for breaths. • **Feel** for breaths on your cheek.
7	If the child is not breathing, give 2 breaths (1 second each). Watch for chest rise as you give each breath.
8	Quickly move or remove clothes from the front of the chest that will get in the way of doing compressions and using an AED.
9	Give 30 compressions at a rate of 100 a minute and then give 2 breaths. After each compression, release pressure on the chest to let it come back to its normal position.
10	After 5 sets of 30 compressions and 2 breaths, if someone has not done this, phone your emergency response number (or 911) and get an AED if available.
11	After you answer all of the dispatcher's questions, return to the child and start the steps of CPR.
12	Keep giving sets of 30 compressions and 2 breaths until an AED arrives, the victim starts to move, or trained help takes over.

Special Situations

When giving CPR to children 1 to 8 years of age, you handle special situations, such as re-opening the airway if the first breath does not go in and the side position, the same way as you do for adults.

1. When giving compressions to a child, press down _____ to _____ the depth of the chest.

2. True or false: If you are alone with a child who does not respond, you should give 5 sets of 30 compressions and 2 breaths before phoning your emergency response number (or 911).

Use of Mask–Adult/Child

Using a Mask

During CPR there is very little chance that you will catch a disease. Some regulatory agencies, including the Occupational Safety and Health Administration (OSHA), require that certain rescuers use a mask when giving breaths in the workplace (Figure 11). You may also want to use a mask or other barrier device when giving CPR to victims outside the workplace who are not family members.

Masks are made of firm plastic and fit over the victim's mouth or mouth and nose. You may need to put the mask together before you use it.

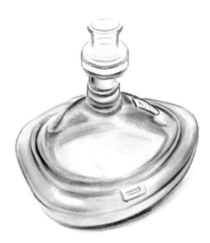

Figure 11. Mask for giving breaths.

Actions for Giving Breaths With a Mask

Follow these steps to give breaths using a mask:

Step	Action
1	Kneel at the victim's side.
2	Put the mask over the victim's mouth and nose.
3	Tilt the head and lift the chin while pressing the mask against the victim's face. It is important to make an airtight seal between the victim's face and the mask while you lift the chin to keep the airway open.
4	Give 2 breaths. Watch for chest rise as you give each breath (Figure 12).

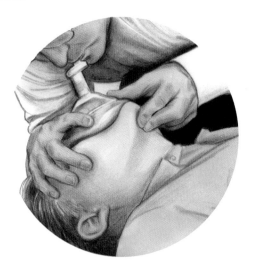

Figure 12. Giving breaths with a mask.

FYI: Masks With Pointed Ends

If the mask has a pointed end

- Put the narrow end of the mask at the top (bridge) of the nose.
- The wide end should cover the mouth.

Adult/Child Choking

What You Will Learn

By the end of this section you should be able to

- List the signs of choking
- Show how to help a choking victim 1 year of age and older

Signs and Actions for Choking

When food or an object such as a toy gets in the airway, it can block the airway. Adults and children can easily choke while eating. Children can also easily choke when playing with small toys.

Choking can be a frightening emergency. If the block in the airway is severe, you must act quickly to remove the block. If you do, you can help the victim breathe.

If the victim	Then the block in the airway is	And you should
• Can make sounds • Can cough loudly	Mild	• Stand by and let the victim cough • If you are worried about the victim's breathing, phone your emergency response number (or 911)
• Cannot breathe • Has a cough that is very quiet or has no sound • Cannot talk or make a sound • Cannot cry (younger child) • Has high-pitched, noisy breathing • Has bluish lips or skin • Makes the choking sign	Severe	• Act quickly • Follow the steps below

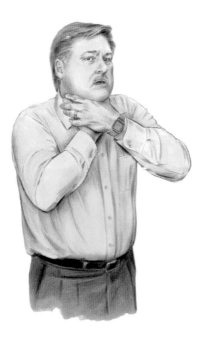

Figure 13. The choking sign. The victim
holds his neck with one or both hands.

How to Help a Choking Victim Over 1 Year of Age

When a victim is choking and suddenly cannot breathe, talk, or make any
sounds, give abdominal thrusts. These thrusts are sometimes called the
Heimlich maneuver. Abdominal thrusts push air from the lungs like a cough.
This can help remove an object blocking the airway. You should give abdominal
thrusts until the object is forced out and the victim can breathe, cough, or talk
or until the victim stops responding.

Follow these steps to help a choking person who is 1 year of age and older:

Step	Action
1	If you think someone is choking, ask, "Are you choking?" If he nods, tell him you are going to help.
2	Kneel or stand firmly behind him and wrap your arms around him so that your hands are in front.
3	Make a fist with one hand.
4	Put the thumb side of your fist slightly above his navel (belly button) and well below the breastbone.
5	Grasp the fist with your other hand and give quick upward thrusts into his abdomen (Figure 14).
6	Give thrusts until the object is forced out and he can breathe, cough, or talk or until he stops responding.

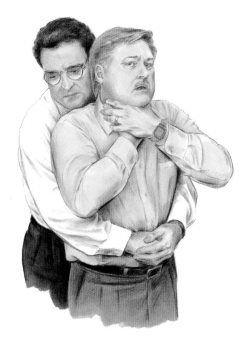

Figure 14. Give quick upward abdominal thrusts.

Important

Encourage all choking victims who have received abdominal thrusts to contact their healthcare provider.

Actions for a Choking Person Who Stops Responding

If you cannot remove the object, the victim will stop responding. When the victim stops responding, follow these steps:

Step	Action
1	Yell for help. If someone comes, send that person to phone your emergency response number (or 911) and get the AED if available.
2	Lower the victim to the ground, faceup. • If you are alone with the adult victim, phone your emergency response number (or 911) and get the AED. Then return to the victim and start the steps of CPR. • If you are alone with the child victim, start the steps of CPR.
3	Every time you open the airway to give breaths, open the victim's mouth wide and look for the object (Figure 15). If you see an object, remove it with your fingers. If you do not see an object, keep giving sets of 30 compressions and 2 breaths until an AED arrives, the victim starts to move, or trained help takes over.
4	After about 5 cycles or 2 minutes, if you are alone, leave the child victim to call your emergency response number (or 911) and get the AED if available.

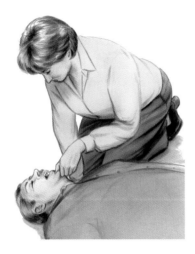

Figure 15. Open the victim's mouth wide and look for the object.

FYI: Asking a Victim About Choking

Sometimes a victim is too young or cannot answer your question for some other reason.

If the adult or child victim does not respond or cannot answer and you think the victim is choking, give abdominal thrusts until the object is forced out and the victim can breathe, cough, or talk or until the victim stops responding.

Actions to Help a Choking Large Person or Pregnant Woman

If the choking victim is in the late stages of pregnancy or is very large, use chest thrusts instead of abdominal thrusts (Figure 16).

Follow the same steps as above except for where you place your arms and hands. Put your arms under the victim's armpits and your hands on the center of the victim's chest. Pull straight back to give the chest thrusts.

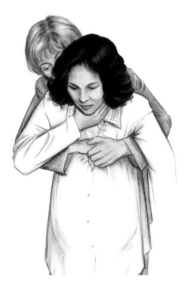

Figure 16. Chest thrusts on a choking large person or pregnant woman.

1. How can you help relieve choking in an adult who is responding but cannot talk?

    a. Back slaps

    b. Nothing

    c. Abdominal thrusts

2. True or false: You should give abdominal thrusts to an adult who is coughing loudly.

Using AEDs

What You Will Learn

By the end of this section you should be able to

- Tell what an AED does
- Tell when you might use an AED
- List the steps for using an AED
- Tell how to give CPR and use an AED

Overview

AEDs are accurate and easy to use. After very little training, most people can operate an AED. Giving CPR right away and using an AED within a few minutes will increase the chances of saving the life of someone with sudden cardiac arrest.

What an AED Does

An automated external defibrillator (AED) is a machine with a computer inside (Figure 17). An AED can

- Recognize cardiac arrest that requires a shock
- Tell the rescuer when a shock is needed
- Give a shock if needed

An AED may give an electric shock to the heart. This can stop the abnormal heart rhythm and allow a normal heart rhythm to return.

The AED will use visual and audible prompts to tell the rescuer the steps to take. There are many different brands of AEDs, but the same simple steps operate all of them.

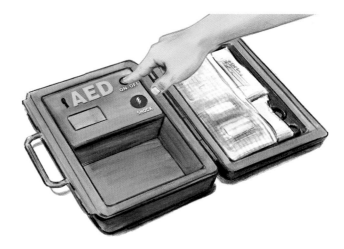

Figure 17. An automated external defibrillator (AED).

When You Might Use an AED

A victim who does not respond may have an abnormal heart rhythm that stops the heart from pumping blood. You will use an AED on a victim 1 year of age and older only when that victim does not respond and is not breathing.

- For victims 8 years of age and older, start CPR right away and use an AED as soon as it is available.

- For victims 1 to 8 years of age, perform 5 sets of 30 compressions and 2 breaths or about 2 minutes of CPR before attaching and using the AED.

FYI: AED Pads

Some AEDs can deliver a smaller shock dose for children if you use child pads or a child key or switch. If the AED can deliver this smaller shock dose, use it for children 1 to 8 years of age. If the AED cannot give a child dose, you can use the adult pads and give an adult shock dose for children 1 to 8 years of age.

For victims 8 years of age and older, always use the larger adult pads and adult dose—DO NOT use child pads or a child dose for a victim 8 years of age and older. You should know how to operate the AED in your workplace and know if it can provide a child dose and how to deliver that dose for a child.

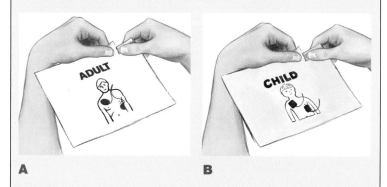

A   B

Figure 18. AED pads. **A,** Adult pads. **B,** Child pads.

For more information on choosing the AED pads or system, refer to the CD.

Steps for Using an AED

Use the same simple steps to operate all AEDs:

Step	Action
1	**Turn the AED on.** Push the button or open the lid (Figure 19). Follow the visual and audible prompts.
2	**Attach pads** (Figure 20).
3	**Allow the AED to check the heart rhythm.** Make sure no one touches the victim (Figure 21).
4	**Push the SHOCK button if the AED tells you to do so** (Figure 22). Make sure no one touches the victim. If a shock is delivered, start the steps of CPR right after shock delivery.

Use the AED fast. For adult victims the time from arrival of the AED to first shock should be less than 90 seconds.

If the AED does not tell you to give a shock, follow the AED visual and audible prompts. Be ready to resume CPR if needed.

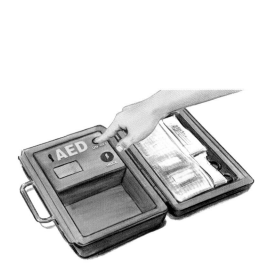

Figure 19. Turn on the AED.

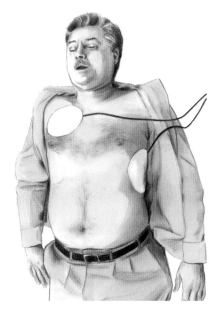

Figure 20. Attach pads.

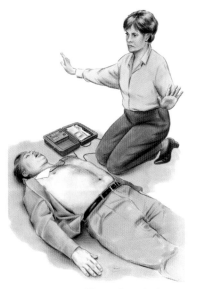

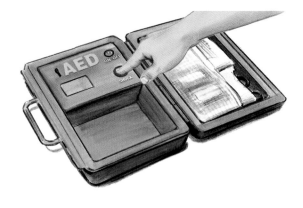

Figure 21. Clear the victim.   **Figure 22.** Press SHOCK button if needed.

Attaching Pads

Follow these steps when attaching pads:

Step	Action
1	Choose the correct pad (adult vs child) for size/age of victim.
2	Open the AED pad package and peel away the plastic backing.
3	Attach the sticky side of the pads directly to the victim's bare chest. The picture on the pad will show you where to put the pads.

Clearing the Victim

You must "clear" the victim before the AED analyzes the victim's heart rhythm or gives a shock dose to the victim. To clear the victim, look around to make sure no one touches the victim when the AED prompts you to clear (Figure 21).

Special Situations

Special situations will change the way you use an AED.

Water
Do not deliver a shock when a victim is

- Lying in water
- Covered with water (for example, the victim is covered with sweat or has just been pulled from a swimming pool)

Water may cause the shock to flow over the skin from one pad to the other. If that happens, energy won't go to the heart.

If you give a shock in water, the AED also might shock the rescuer.

Step	Action
1	Move the victim away from standing water.
2	Quickly wipe the victim's chest before you attach the pads.

FYI: AEDs and Small Amounts of Water

If the victim is lying in a small puddle of water or snow but the chest is not covered with water, you can give shocks.

Medicine Patch

You should not put an AED pad over a medicine patch. The patch may block some of the shock dose so that some of the energy does not reach the heart. Also, giving a shock over the patch may burn the victim.

Step	Action
1	If a child or adult has a medicine patch in the same place where you would attach the AED pad, take the medicine patch off while wearing gloves.
2	Quickly wipe the chest where the patch was before you put on the pad.

Implanted Pacemaker or Defibrillator

Some children or adults may have an implanted pacemaker or defibrillator. These devices make a hard lump under the skin of the chest or in the abdomen. The lump is smaller than a deck of cards. You should not put an AED pad over this lump because the implanted device may block delivery of the shock to the heart.

Step	Action
1	Look for a lump under the skin of the chest that looks smaller than a deck of cards.
2	If you see this lump where the pads should go, put the pads at least 1 inch away from the lump.

Hairy Chest

If a victim has a hairy chest, the AED pads may stick to the hair instead of the skin on the chest. If this happens, the AED will not be able to check the victim's heart rhythm or deliver a shock. The AED will prompt you to check the pads.

Step	Action
1	If the pads stick to the hair instead of the skin, press down firmly on each pad.
2	If the AED still tells you to check the pads, quickly pull off the pads to remove the hair.
3	If a lot of hair still remains where you will put the pads, shave the area with the razor in the AED carrying case.
4	Put on a new set of pads. Follow the AED visual and audible prompts.

FYI: AEDs in the Community

The American Heart Association supports placing AEDs throughout the community in lay rescuer AED programs. AEDs are placed in many public places where large numbers of people gather, such as sports stadiums, airports, airplanes, and an increasing number of worksites.

AED programs usually are directed by a healthcare provider and are linked with the local EMS system. AED rescuers, such as police, security guards, trained first aid providers, and volunteers should be trained in CPR and the use of an AED.

You can increase the chance of survival for a victim of sudden cardiac arrest if you give the victim CPR right away and use an AED within a few minutes.

For more information on taking care of an AED, refer to the CD.

Notes

You can get the answers for these items at your workplace after the course.

Key Points From My Workplace Emergency Response Policies and Procedures

How to access the workplace emergency response system:

Phone:_____

Where the AED (if avaliable) is located: _____

What changes do you need to make to use the AED on a child?

____Use "child" pads

____Insert a "child" key or turn a "child" switch

____Other: _____

Masks used at the workplace (check one):

____Yes ____ No

Other key points:

_____

_____

_____

Review Questions

1. True or false: You can use adult AED pads on a child if child pads are not available.

2. Which of the following best describes "clearing the victim"?

   a. Taking the pads off the victim's chest
   b. Making sure no one is touching the victim
   c. Moving the victim to a clear room

Infant CPR

What You Will Learn	By the end of this section you should be able to give CPR to an infant.
Ages for Infant CPR	Infant CPR is for victims from birth to 1 year of age.
Overview	Although some steps for giving CPR to an infant are similar to giving CPR to an adult or child, there are a few differences:

- How to give compressions
- How to open the airway
- How to give breaths
- How to use a mask
- How to check for response

You will first learn the skills of CPR for the infant that are different from adult and child CPR. Then you will learn to put all the steps together in the correct order.

Compressions	As with CPR for the adult and child, compressions are a very important part of infant CPR. Compressions pump blood to the brain and heart.
Actions for Compressions	Follow these steps to give compressions to an infant:

Step	Action
1	Place the infant on a firm, flat surface. If possible, place the infant on a surface above the ground, such as a table. This makes it easier to give CPR to the infant.
2	Quickly move or open clothes from the front of the chest that will get in the way of doing compressions.
3	Put 2 fingers of one hand just below the nipple line. Do not put your fingers over the very bottom of the breastbone (Figure 23).
4	Press the infant's breastbone straight down ⅓ to ½ *the depth* of the chest. Push hard and fast.
5	Repeat at a rate of 100 compressions a minute.
6	After each compression, release pressure on the chest to let it come back to its normal position.

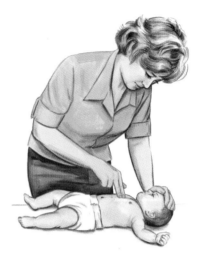

Figure 23. Put 2 fingers just below the nipple line.

> ### *Important*
>
> These things are important to remember when doing CPR:
>
> - Push hard and push fast.
> - Push at a rate of 100 times a minute.
> - After each compression, release pressure on the chest to let it come back to its normal position.

Open the Airway

When giving CPR, you must give the infant breaths that make the chest rise. Before giving breaths you must open the airway with the head tilt–chin lift.

Performing the Head Tilt–Chin Lift

When you open an infant's airway, use the head tilt–chin lift (Figure 24). When tilting an infant's head, do not push it back too far because it may block the infant's airway.

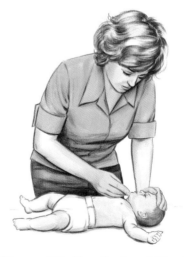

Figure 24. Use the head tilt–chin lift.

Giving Breaths

Breaths are very important for infants who are not breathing or do not respond. Your breaths give an infant oxygen when the infant cannot breathe on his own. You will not have to give as large a breath to an infant as you give to a child or an adult.

Actions for Giving Breaths

Follow these steps to give breaths to infants:

Step	Action
1	Hold the infant's airway open with a head tilt–chin lift.
2	Take a normal breath and cover the infant's mouth and nose with your mouth, creating an airtight seal (Figure 25).
3	Give 2 breaths (blow for 1 second each). Watch for chest rise as you give each breath.

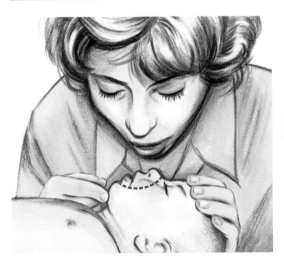

Figure 25. Cover the infant's mouth and nose with your mouth.

FYI: Tips for Giving Breaths

If your mouth is too small to cover the infant's mouth and nose, put your mouth over the infant's nose and give breaths through the infant's nose. (You may need to hold the infant's mouth closed to prevent air from escaping through the mouth.)

Check for Response

Check to see if the infant responds before giving CPR. Tap the infant's foot and shout, "Are you OK?" (Figure 26).

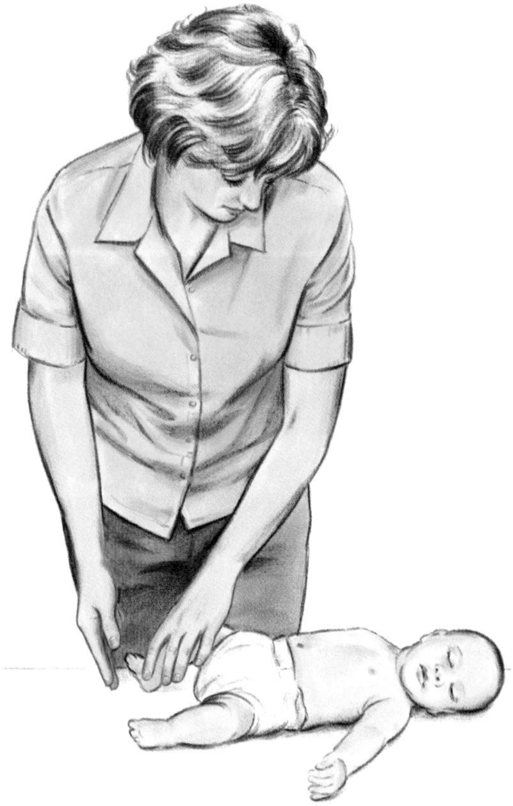

Figure 26. Check for response.

Get Help

If the infant does not respond, it is important to get help on the way as soon as possible. Follow these steps to get help:

Step	Action
1	If the infant does not respond, yell for help. If someone comes, send that person to phone your emergency response number (or 911).
2	If no one comes, stay with the infant and continue the steps of CPR.

Special Situation

If you give an infant a breath and it does not go in, you will need to re-open the airway with a head tilt–chin lift before giving the second breath.

Summary of Steps for Infant CPR

The following table summarizes the steps for infant CPR:

Step	Action
1	Make sure the scene is safe.
2	Tap the infant's foot and shout to see if the infant responds.
3	If the infant does not respond, yell for help. • If someone comes, send that person to phone your emergency response number (or 911). • If no one comes, stay with the infant to start the steps of CPR.
4	Place the infant on a firm, flat surface. If possible, place the infant on a surface above the ground, such as a table.
5	Open the airway with a head tilt–chin lift.
6	Check to see if the infant is breathing (take at least 5 seconds but no more than 10 seconds). • Put your ear next to the infant's mouth and nose. • **Look** to see if the chest rises. • **Listen** for breaths. • **Feel** for breaths on your cheek.
7	If the infant is not breathing, give 2 breaths (1 second each). Watch for chest rise as you give each breath.
8	Quickly move or open clothes from the front of the chest that will get in the way of doing compressions.
9	Give 30 compressions at a rate of 100 a minute and then give 2 breaths. After each compression, release pressure on the chest to let it come back to its normal position.
10	After 5 sets of 30 compressions and 2 breaths, if someone has not done this, leave the infant and phone your emergency response number (or 911).
11	After you answer all of the dispatcher's questions, return to the infant and start the steps of CPR.
12	Keep giving sets of 30 compressions and 2 breaths until the infant starts to move or trained help takes over.

> ### FYI: Taking the Infant With You to Phone for Help
>
> If the infant is not injured and you are alone, after 5 sets of 30 compressions and 2 breaths, you may carry the infant with you to phone your emergency response number (or 911).

Review Questions

1. The correct rate for giving compressions is _____ compressions a minute.

2. For infant CPR you give sets of _____ compressions and _____ breaths.

3. When giving CPR to an infant, how long should each breath take?

   a. 1 second

   b. 3 seconds

   c. 4 seconds

Use of Mask–Infant

Using a Mask

Using a mask for an infant is the same as for an adult or child except for a couple of things:

- Any mask should cover the infant's nose and mouth but should not cover the infant's eyes.

- If you do not have an infant mask, follow the recommendations of the manufacturer of the mask you are using.

Infant Choking

| **What You Will Learn** | By the end of this section you should be able to show how to help a choking infant. |

Signs of Choking

When food or an object such as a toy gets in the airway, it can block the airway. Infants can easily choke if they put small things in their mouths.

Choking can be a frightening emergency. If the block in the airway is severe, you must act quickly to remove the block. If you do, you can help the infant breathe.

The signs of choking are the same for adults, children, and infants except that the infant will not use the choking sign.

How to Help a Choking Infant

When an infant is choking and suddenly cannot breathe or make any sounds, you must act quickly to help get the object out by using back slaps and chest thrusts.

Follow these steps to relieve choking in an infant:

Step	Action
1	Hold the infant facedown on your forearm. Support the infant's head and jaw with your hand. Sit or kneel and rest your arm on your lap or thigh.
2	Give up to 5 back slaps with the heel of your free hand between the infant's shoulder blades (Figure 27).
3	If the object does not come out after 5 back slaps, turn the infant onto his back. Move or open the clothes from the front of the chest only if you can do so quickly. You can push on the chest through clothes if you need to.
4	Give up to 5 chest thrusts using 2 fingers of your free hand to push on the breastbone in the same place you push for compressions (Figure 28). • Support the head and neck. • Hold the infant with one hand and arm, resting your arm on your lap or thigh.
5	Alternate giving 5 back slaps and 5 chest thrusts until the object comes out and the infant can breathe, cough, or cry, or until the infant stops responding.

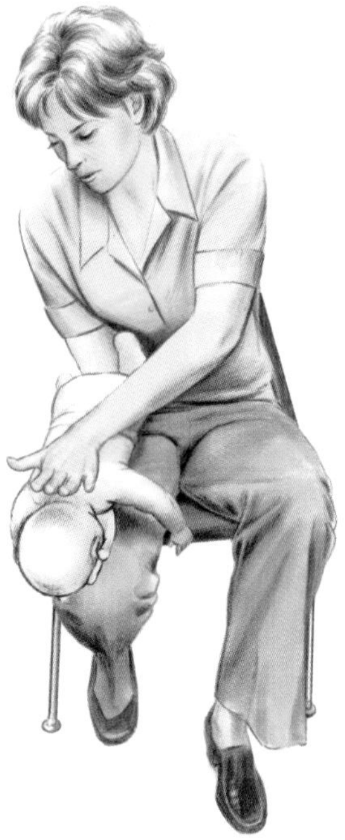

Figure 27. Give up to 5 back slaps with the heel of your hand.

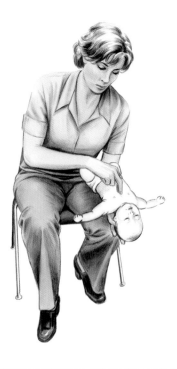

Figure 28. Give up to 5 chest thrusts.

When to Stop Back Slaps and Chest Thrusts

Stop back slaps and chest thrusts if

- The object comes out
- The infant begins to breathe, cough, or cry
- The infant stops responding

Actions for a Choking Infant Who Stops Responding

If you cannot remove the object, the infant will stop responding. When the infant stops responding, follow these steps:

Step	Action
1	Yell for help. If someone comes, send that person to phone your emergency response number (or 911). Stay with the infant to start the steps of CPR.
2	Place the infant on a firm, flat surface. If possible, place the infant on a surface above the ground, such as a table.
3	Start the steps of CPR.
4	Every time you open the airway to give breaths, open the infant's mouth wide and look for the object. If you see an object, remove it with your fingers. If you do not see an object, keep giving sets of 30 compressions and 2 breaths. Continue CPR until the infant starts to move or trained help takes over.
5	After about 5 cycles or 2 minutes, if you are alone, leave the infant to call your emergency response number (or 911).
6	Return to the infant and continue the steps of CPR.

Do Not

DO NOT use abdominal thrusts on an infant. Abdominal thrusts could injure an infant.

Review Questions

1. How can you help relieve choking in an infant who is responding and crying?
   a. Back slaps and chest thrusts
   b. Nothing
   c. Abdominal thrusts

2. True or false: You should try to relieve choking if an infant is coughing loudly.

Phoning for Help

PHONING FOR HELP

What You Will Learn

By the end of this section you should be able to

- Tell how to phone your emergency response number (or 911)
- Tell how to answer a dispatcher's questions

Access to Emergency Medical Service

At times you will need to phone your emergency response number (or 911) for help. Make sure you know your phone system. Do you need to dial 9 or another number to get an outside line before you dial your emergency response number (or 911)? Know this *before* you need to phone for help.

Keep emergency numbers near or on the telephone(s), including your emergency response number and Poison Control (800-222-1222).

Your Emergency Response Number

If there is an emergency in this area, phone _____ (fill in the blank).

Phoning for Help

This section includes general guidelines for phoning for help. Your organization may have specific rules about when you should phone your emergency response number. Make sure you know your organization's rules.

Reasons to Phone for Help

As a general rule, you should phone your emergency response number (or 911) and ask for help whenever

- Someone is seriously ill or hurt
- You are not sure what to do in an emergency

Remember: It is better to phone for help even if you might not need it than not to phone when someone does need help.

Answering Dispatcher Questions

When you phone your emergency response number (or 911), the dispatcher will ask you some questions about the emergency. You need to stay on the phone until the dispatcher tells you to hang up. The dispatcher can also tell you how to help the victim until trained help takes over.

45

Review Questions

1. My emergency response number is _____.

2. True or false: You should phone your emergency response number (or 911) and ask for help whenever someone is seriously ill or hurt.

Conclusion

Congratulations on taking time to attend this course. Contact the American Heart Association if you want more information on CPR, AEDs, or even first aid. You can visit *www.americanheart.org/cpr* or call 877-AHA-4CPR (877-242-4277) to find a class near you.

Even if you don't remember all the steps of CPR exactly, it is important for you to try. And always remember to phone your emergency response number (or 911). They can remind you what to do.

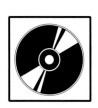

For information on signs of heart attack and stroke, as well as general anatomy and physiology, refer to the CD.

CONCLUSION

Comparison of CPR and AED Steps
for Adults, Children, and Infants

CPR	Adult and Older Child (8 Years of Age and Older)	Child (1 to 8 Years Old)	Infant (Less Than 1 Year Old)
Check for response	Tap and shout		Tap the infant's foot and shout
Phone your emergency response number (or 911)	Phone your emergency response number (or 911) as soon as you find that the victim does not respond	Phone your emergency response number (or 911) after giving 5 sets of 30 compressions and 2 breaths	
Open the airway Use head tilt–chin lift	Head tilt–chin lift		Head tilt–chin lift (do not tilt head back too far)
Check breathing If the victim is not breathing, give 2 breaths that make the chest rise	Open the airway, look, listen, and feel (Take at least 5 seconds but no more than 10 seconds)		
First 2 breaths	Give 2 breaths (1 second each)		
Start CPR	Give sets of 30 compressions and 2 breaths		
• **Compression location**	Center of chest between nipples		Just below the nipple line
• **Compression method**	2 hands	1 or 2 hands	2 fingers
• **Compression depth**	1½ to 2 inches	⅓ to ½ depth of chest	
• **Compression rate**	100 a minute		
• **Sets of compressions and breaths**	30:2		
To relieve choking	Abdominal thrusts		Back slaps and chest thrusts (no abdominal thrusts)
AED • **Turn the power on (or open the case)**	Use AED as soon as it arrives	Use AED after 5 sets of 30 compressions and 2 breaths	
• **Attach pads to the victim's bare chest**	Use adult pads	Use child pads/key/switch or adult pads	
• **Allow the AED to check the heart rhythm**	Clear and analyze		
• **Push the SHOCK button if prompted by the AED**	Clear and shock		
• **Time from arrival of AED to first shock**	Less than 90 seconds		

Heartsaver AED Course
Adult/Child CPR and AED
Student Practice Sheet

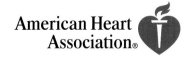

American Heart Association®

Learn and Live ℠

Step	Critical Performance Steps	Details
1	_____ Check for response	Tap victim and ask if the person is "all right" or "OK," speaking loudly and clearly.
2	_____ Tell someone to phone your emergency response number (or 911) and get an AED	Tell someone to perform **both** actions.
3	_____ Open airway using head tilt–chin lift	Place palm of one hand on forehead. Place fingers of other hand under the lower jaw to lift the chin. Obvious movement of the head back toward the hand on the forehead.
4	_____ Check breathing	Place face near the victim's nose and mouth to listen and feel for victim's breath. Look at chest. Take at least 5 seconds but no more than 10 seconds.
5	_____ Give 2 breaths (1 second each)	Seal your mouth over victim's mouth and blow. Your exhaled breaths should take 1 second each. Reposition the head if chest does not rise.
6	_____ Bare victim's chest and locate CPR hand position	Move or remove clothing from front of victim's chest. Place heel of one hand in the center of chest, between the nipples.
7	_____ Deliver first cycle of 30 compressions at the correct rate	Give 30 compressions in less than 23 seconds. Push hard; push fast; let chest return to normal between compressions.
8	_____ Give 2 breaths (1 second each)	Seal your mouth over victim's mouth and blow. Your exhaled breaths should take 1 second each. Reposition the head if chest does not rise.

PRACTICE SHEETS

Step	Critical Performance Steps	Details
AED Arrives		
AED 1	_____ Turn AED on	Stop CPR and press button to turn AED on (or make sure that AED case is open if your AED has an automatic-on feature).
AED 2	_____ Select proper pads and place pads correctly	Recognize the difference between adult pads and child pads: • Select the proper pad size for the manikin • Apply the pads to the chest as pad diagrams and/or AED instructions show
AED 3	_____ Clear victim to analyze	Show a visible sign of clearing the victim and a spoken indication of clearing the victim: "Clear! Stay clear of victim!" or similar words with an obvious gesture to make sure all are clear.
AED 4	_____ Clear victim to shock/press shock button	Show a visible sign of clearing the victim and a spoken indication of clearing the victim: "Clear! Stay clear of victim!" or similar words with an obvious gesture to make sure all are clear. Press shock button when prompted and after clearing. For adult victim, time from arrival of AED to first shock must be less than 90 seconds.
Continue CPR		
9	_____ Resume CPR: deliver second cycle of compressions using correct hand position	Place heel of one hand in the center of chest, between the nipples. Do 30 compressions. Push hard; push fast; let chest return to normal between compressions.
10	_____ Give 2 breaths (1 second each)	Seal your mouth over victim's mouth and blow. Your exhaled breaths should take 1 second each. Reposition the head if chest does not rise.
11	_____ Deliver third cycle of compressions of adequate depth with chest returning to normal	Do 30 compressions. Push hard; push fast; let chest return to normal between compressions.

Heartsaver AED Course
Infant CPR
Student Practice Sheet

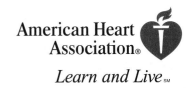

American Heart Association®

Learn and Live ℠

Step	Critical Performance Steps	Details
1	_____ Check for response	Tap infant's foot and shout loudly.
2	_____ Tell someone to phone your emergency response number (or 911)	Tell someone to phone emergency response number (or 911). (During class practice there is someone to phone 911; otherwise do 2 minutes of CPR before phoning 911.)
3	_____ Open airway using head tilt–chin lift	Push back on forehead, place fingers on the bony part of the victim's chin and lift the victim's chin. Do not press the neck or under the chin. Lift the jaw upward by bringing the chin forward. Do not push the head back too far.
4	_____ Check breathing	Place face near the victim's nose and mouth to listen and feel for victim's breath. Look at chest. Take at least 5 seconds but no more than 10 seconds.
5	_____ Give 2 breaths (1 second each) with visible chest rise	Seal your mouth over victim's nose and mouth and blow. Your exhaled breaths should take 1 second each. You should be able to see the chest rise twice.
6	_____ Bare victim's chest and locate CPR finger position	Move or open clothing from front of victim's chest. Place 2 fingers just below the nipple line.
7	_____ Deliver first cycle of 30 compressions at the correct rate	Give 30 compressions in less than 23 seconds. Push hard; push fast; let chest return to normal between compressions.
8	_____ Give 2 breaths (1 second each) with visible chest rise	Seal your mouth over victim's nose and mouth and blow. Your exhaled breaths should take 1 second each. You should be able to see the chest rise twice.
9	_____ Deliver second cycle of compressions using correct finger position	Compress chest with 2 fingers just below the nipple line. Do 30 compressions. Push hard; push fast; let chest return to normal between compressions.
10	_____ Give 2 breaths (1 second each) with visible chest rise	Seal your mouth over victim's nose and mouth and blow. Your exhaled breaths should take 1 second each. You should be able to see the chest rise twice.
11	_____ Deliver third cycle of compressions of adequate depth with chest returning to normal	Do 30 compressions. Push hard; push fast; let chest return to normal between compressions.

Heartsaver AED Course Evaluation

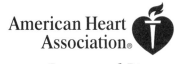

American Heart
Association®

Learn and Live SM

Our goal is to ensure that we are providing an effective program that meets your needs and expectations. We value your opinion and need your feedback. Please take a moment to complete this course evaluation. The administrator of this program will review your ratings and comments on the delivery, facilities, instructor, and overall satisfaction with the course.

Administration and Facilities

Date of course? _____ Who were the instructors? _____

Where was the course held? _____

Circle a number that matches your opinion on each statement.	Strongly Disagree	Disagree	Neutral	Agree	Strongly Agree
It was easy to enroll in the course.	1	2	3	4	5
I received my *Heartsaver Student Workbook* and CD in time for me to read the pre-class assignments.	1	2	3	4	5
The course facilities were adequate.	1	2	3	4	5
There was enough equipment available for everyone to practice skills with little "standing around" time.	1	2	3	4	5
The equipment was clean and in good working order.	1	2	3	4	5

Instruction

Circle a number that matches your opinion on each statement.	Strongly Disagree	Disagree	Neutral	Agree	Strongly Agree
My instructor communicated clearly.	1	2	3	4	5
My instructor answered my questions.	1	2	3	4	5

Satisfaction

Circle a number that matches your opinion on each statement.	Strongly Disagree	Disagree	Neutral	Agree	Strongly Agree
I would recommend this course to others.	1	2	3	4	5
I can apply the skills I learned.	1	2	3	4	5

Any comments you would like to make on the delivery, facilities, instructor, and overall satisfaction with the course? Please write your comments on the back of this form.

Please return your completed course evaluation to your instructor or your regional ECC office.